My Lean and Gree

Diet Pla..

50 super easy and affordable lean and green breakfast recipes to burn fat fast and start the day

Josephine Reed

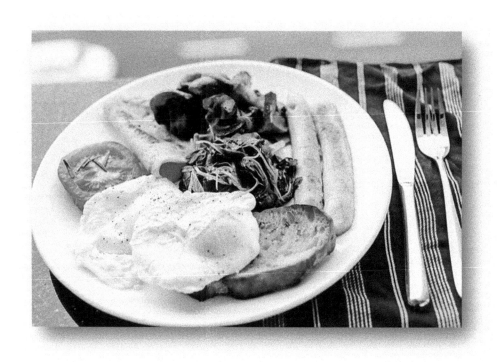

Please consult a licensed professional before attempting any techniques outlined in this book.

By reading this document, the reader agrees that under no circumstances is the author responsible for any losses, direct or indirect, which are incurred as a result of the use of information contained within this document, including, but not limited to, — errors, omissions, or inaccuracies.

Table of contents

Barley Risotto

Prep Time: 15 minutes

Cook Time: 7 to 8 hours

Serve: 8

Ingredients:

- 21/4 cups hulled barley, rinsed

- 1 onion, finely chopped

- 4 garlic cloves, minced

- 1 (8-ounce) package button mushrooms, chopped

- 6 cups low-sodium vegetable broth

- 1/2 teaspoon dried marjoram leaves

- 1/8 teaspoon freshly ground black pepper

- 2/3 cup grated Parmesan cheese

Instructions:

1. In a 6-quart slow cooker, mix the barley, onion, garlic, mushrooms, broth, marjoram, and pepper.

2. Cook for 7/8 hours or until most of the liquid is absorbed and tender and the vegetables are tender, or until the barley is full.

3. Stir in the Parmesan cheese and serve.

Nutrition: Calories: 288 Cal, Carbohydrates: 45 g, Sugar: 2 g, Fiber: 9 g, Fat: 6 g, Saturated Fat: 3 g, Protein: 13 g, Sodium: 495 mg

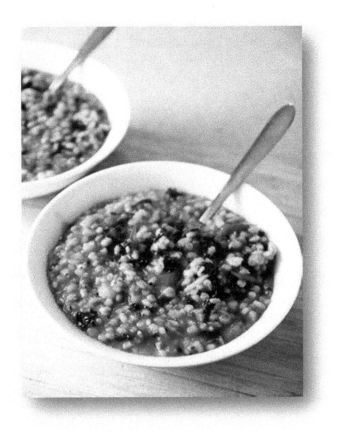

Risotto with Green Beans, Sweet Potatoes, and Peas

Prep Time: 20 minutes

Cook Time: 4 to 5 hours

Serve: 8

Ingredients:

- 1 large sweet potato, peeled and chopped

- 1 onion, chopped

- 5 garlic cloves, minced

- 2 cups short-grain brown rice

- 1 teaspoon dried thyme leaves

- 7 cups low-sodium vegetable broth

- 2 cups green beans, cut in half crosswise

- 2 cups frozen baby peas

- 3 tablespoons unsalted butter

- 1/2 cup grated Parmesan cheese

Instructions:

1. In a 6-quart slow cooker, mix the sweet potato, onion, garlic, rice, thyme, and broth.

2. Cook on low heat for 3/4 hours, or until the rice is tender.

3. Stir in the green beans and frozen peas.

4. Cook on low heat for 30 to 40 minutes or until the vegetables are tender.

5. Stir in the butter and cheese. Cook for 20 minutes over low heat, then stir and serve.

Nutrition: Calories: 385 Cal, Carbohydrates: 52 g, Sugar: 4 g, Fiber: 6 g, Fat: 10 g, Saturated Fat: 5 g, Protein: 10 g, Sodium: 426 mg

Prawn Arrabbiata

Prep Time: 35 minutes

Cook Time: 30 minutes

Serve: 1

Ingredients:

- Raw or cooked prawns, 1 cup

- Extra virgin olive oil, 1 tablespoon

- Buckwheat pasta, ½ cup

- Chopped parsley, 1 tablespoon

- Celery, ¼ cup (finely chopped)

- Tinned chopped tomatoes, 2 cups

- Red onion, 1/3 cup (finely chopped)

- Garlic clove, 1 (finely chopped)

- Extra virgin olive oil, 1 teaspoon

- Dried mixed herbs, 1 teaspoon

- Bird's eye chili, 1 (finely chopped)

- White wine, 2 tablespoons (optional)

Instructions:

1. Add the olive oil into your fry-pan and fry the dried herbs, celery, and onions over medium-low heat for about two minutes.

2. Increase the heat to low, add the wine and simmer for another minute.

3. Add the tomatoes to the pan and allow to simmer for about 30 minutes, over medium-low heat, until you get a good creamy consistency, over medium-low heat.

4. If the sauce gets too thick, add a bit of water.

5. Cook the pasta while the sauce is heating, following the packet's instructions. Drain the water once the pasta is done cooking, toss with the olive oil, and set aside until needed.

6. If using raw prawns, add them to your sauce and cook for another four minutes, until the prawns turn opaque and pink, then add the parsley. If using cooked prawns, add them at the same time with the parsley and allow the sauce to boil.

7. Add the already cooked pasta to the sauce, mix them, and serve.

Nutrition: Calories: 321, Protein: 19 g, Fat: 2 g, Carbohydrate: 23 g

Mediterranean Baked Penne

Prep Time: 25 minutes

Cook Time: 1 hour 20 minutes

Serve: 8

Ingredients:

- Extra-virgin olive oil, 1 tablespoon

- Fine dry breadcrumbs, ½ cup

- Small zucchini, 2 (chopped)

- Medium eggplant, 1 (chopped)

- Medium onion, 1 (chopped)

- Red bell pepper, 1 (seeded and chopped)

- Celery, 1 stalk (sliced)

- Garlic, 1 clove (minced)

- Salt and freshly ground pepper to taste

- Dry white wine, ¼ cup

- Plum tomatoes, 28-ounces (drained and coarsely chopped, juice reserved)

- Freshly grated Parmesan cheese, 2 tablespoons

- Large eggs, 2 (lightly beaten)

- Coarsely grated part-skim mozzarella cheese, 1 ½ cups

- Dried penne rig ate or rigatoni, 1 pound

Instructions:

1. Preheat to 375 degrees F in your oven. Apply nonstick spray on a 3-quart baking dish. Then coat the dish with ¼ cup of breadcrumbs, tapping out the excess.

2. Heat the oil in a big non-stick skillet over medium to high heat. Then add the onion, celery, bell pepper, eggplant, and zucchini. Cook, stirring periodically, for about 10 minutes, until smooth.Then add the garlic and cook for another minute. Add the wine, stir and cook for about 2 minutes, long enough for the wine to almost evaporate. Then add the juice and tomatoes. Bring it to a boil for 10/15 minutes or so, until thickened, season with pepper and salt. Put it in a large bowl to let it cool.

3. Pour water into a pot and add some salt when then allow to boil. Add the penne into the boiling salted water to cook for about 10 minutes, until al dente. Drain the pasta under running water and rinse it. Toss the pasta with the vegetable mixture, then stir in the mozzarella.

4. Scoop the pasta mixture and place into the prepared baking dish. Drizzle the broken eggs evenly over the top. Mix the Parmesan and ¼ cups of breadcrumbs in a small bowl, then sprinkle evenly over the top of the dish.

5. Cook the dish in the oven for 40/50 minutes or so, until bubbly and golden.

6. Allow to rest for 10 min before you serve.

Nutrition: Calories: 372, Protein: 45 g, Fat: 8 g, Sugar: 2 g

Jalapeno Cheese Balls

Prep Time: 10 minutes

Cook Time: 8 minutes

Serve: 1

Ingredients:

- 1-ounce cream cheese
- 1/6 cup shredded mozzarella cheese
- 1/6 cup shredded Cheddar cheese
- 1/2 jalapeños, finely chopped
- 1/2 cup breadcrumbs
- Two eggs
- 1/2 cup all-purpose flour
- Salt and Pepper
- Cooking oil

Instructions:

1. Combine the cream cheese, mozzarella, Cheddar, and jalapeños in a medium bowl. Mix well.

2. Form the cheese mixture into balls about an inch thick. You may also use a small ice cream scoop. It works well.

3. Arrange the cheese balls on a sheet pan and place in the freezer for 15 minutes. It will help the cheese balls maintain their shape while frying.

4. Spray the Instant Crisp Air Fryer basket with cooking oil.

5. Place the breadcrumbs in a small bowl. In another small bowl, beat the eggs. In the third small bowl, combine the flour with salt and pepper to taste, and mix well.

6. Remove the cheese balls from the freezer. Plunge the cheese balls in the flour, then the eggs, and then the breadcrumbs.

7. Place the cheese balls in the Instant Crisp Air Fryer. Spray with cooking oil. Lock the air fryer lid. Cook for 8 minutes.

8. Open the Instant Crisp Air Fryer and flip the cheese balls. I recommend flipping them instead of shaking, so the balls maintain their form. Cook an additional 4 minutes.

9. Cool before serving.

Nutrition: Calories: 96, Fat: 6 g, Protein: 4 g, Sugar: 0 g

Chicken with Spinach and Mushrooms

Prep Time: 10 minutes

Cook Time: 20 minutes

Serve: 4

Ingredients:

- 1 tbsp. olive oil

- 4 6-oz boneless, skinless breasts of chicken Black pepper and kosher salt

- 1 lb. quartered button mushrooms

- 1 red-bell-pepper, sliced into 1/2-inch bits 2 garlic cloves, chopped

- One-half cup white dry wine

- 2 bunches of spinach, removal of thick stems (about 8 cups)

Instructions:

1.Heat 1 little-spoon of oil over medium to high heat in a large skillet. With a one-half teaspoon of salt and one-fourth teaspoon of pepper, season the poultry.

2.Cook the chicken, 6 to 7 minutes on each side until browned and cooked through. Move to a dish.

3.Send the skillet back to medium-high heat and heat the remaining oil tablespoon. Cook the mushrooms and pepper for 3 minutes, tossing.

4.Add the garlic and wine and cook for 2 to 3 minutes, until the mushrooms are tender and the wine has almost evaporated.

5.Toss the salt and pepper with the spinach, one-half teaspoon each, and eat with the chicken.

Nutrition: calories: 743 kcal Protein: 32.24 g Fat: 18.27 g Carbohydrates: 129.82 g Calcium, Ca227 mg Magnesium, Mg324 mg

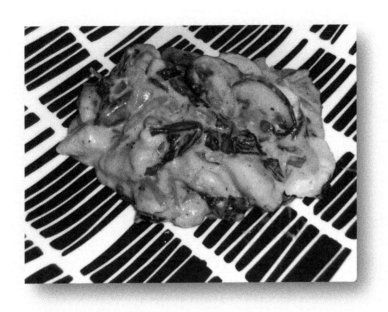

Creamy Pesto Chicken

Prep time: 10 min

Cook Time: 15 min

Serve: 2

Ingredients:

- 1 tablespoon extra virgin olive oil

- 4 chicken breast halves - cut into strips

- 4 large cloves garlic, sliced

- 3 1/2 tablespoons sherry

- 1/4 cup pine nuts

- 1/2 cup chopped fresh basil

- 1 (8 ounces) container reduced-fat sour cream

- 3 tablespoons grated Parmesan cheese

- ground black pepper to taste

Instructions:

1.In a frying contaniner, heat olive oil over medium heat and cook the chicken until turning light brown, about 5 minutes. Stir into the frying pan the sherry and garlic. Stir and cook until the juices run clear, the chicken is not pink anymore, and all the liquid has decreased.

2.Stir into the frying pan the pine nuts, and cook over medium heat for 2-3 minutes. Stir in the pepper, parmesan cheese, sour cream, and basil and lower the heat to mild. Until completely cooked, keep cooking.

Nutrition: Calories 312, Fat 6, Carbs 16, Protein 12, Sodium 645

Gnocchi With Chicken, Pesto And Fresh Mozzarella

Prep time: 10 min

Cook Time: 30 min

Serve: 2

Ingredients:

- 1 tablespoon olive oil

- 1 chicken breast half - cut into 1 1/2-inch cube

- salt and ground black pepper to taste

- 2 tablespoons chicken broth

- 1 (8 ounces) jar prepared pesto

- 1 (12 ounces) package potato gnocchi

- 4 ounces small fresh mozzarella balls

Instructions:

In a saucepan, bring olive oil to heat. Add pepper and salt to chicken pieces to season; cook, stirring, for 7-10 minutes in hot oil until no pink meat remains in the center. With a slotted spoon, bring the chicken to a bowl while reserving drippings in the pan.

24

Add chicken broth into the saucepan. Boil broth, using a wooden spoon to scrape browned bits off the bottom of the pan; keep boiling for another 7-10 minutes until broth is reduced by about half of its original volume. Put cooked chicken back into the saucepan. Whisk in pesto; turn off the heat.

Slightly boil lightly salted water in a large pot. Cook gnocchi for about 3 minutes in boiling water until they float to the top. With a slotted spoon, transfer gnocchi from the water to a big bowl while reserving water in the pot.

Set pesto and chicken saucepan over boiling water; cook, stirring, for about 5minutes above boiling water until completely warmed. Cover gnocchi with warmed pesto-chicken mixture; top with mozzarella and stir until combined evenly.

Nutrition: Calories 464, Fat 12, Carbs 16, Protein 23, Sodium 643

Instant Pot Gourmet Pesto Chicken

Prep time: 10 min

Cook Time: 30 min

Serve: 2

Ingredients:

- 5 bone-in chicken thighs, skinned

- salt and ground black pepper to taste

- 1 tablespoon all-purpose flour, or as needed

- 1 tablespoon olive oil

- 1 1/2 cups chicken broth

- 1 (8 ounces) package cream cheese

- 1 (12 ounces) package penne pasta

- 2 cups cut asparagus, 1-inch lengths

- 2 cups cut green beans, 1-inch pieces

- 4 ounces basil pesto (such as Classico® Traditional)

- 1/4 teaspoon onion powder

- 1/4 teaspoon garlic powder

Instructions:

1.Add salt and pepper to the chicken. Coat with flour and dust off the excess.

2.Turn on a pressure cooker that is multi-functional (such as the Instant Pot ®). Select its "Sauté" function. Add olive oil and chicken. Cook the chicken for about 3 minutes or until very lightly browned. Pour in the chicken broth. Close and lock the lid. Select the "Poultry" setting and set the cooker's timer for 30 minutes. Let the pressure build for about 10 to 15 minutes.

3.Refer to the manufacturer's instructions on the quick-release method and carefully release pressure for about 5 minutes. Carefully unlock and remove the lid.

4.Mix in the garlic powder, cream cheese, green beans, onion powder, penne pasta, pesto, and asparagus. Stir together until well combined. Close the lid, select the "Rice" function, and set the timer for 3 minutes. Let the pressure build for 10 to 15 minutes. Cook according to the manufacturer's instructions.

5.Refer to the manufacturer's instructions on the quick-release method and carefully release pressure for about 5 minutes. Unlock and remove the lid.

Nutrition: Calories 408, Fat 6, Carbs 16, Protein 18, Sodium 308

Italian Chicken With Pesto Potatoes

Prep time: 10 min

Cook Time: 30 min

Serve: 2

Ingredients:

- 3/4 cup balsamic vinegar

- 4 skinless, boneless chicken breast halves

- 4 1/2 ounces sliced mozzarella cheese

- salt and pepper to taste

- 4 slices Parma ham

- 1-pint cherry tomatoes

- 1 tablespoon olive oil

- 1 pound small potatoes

- 2 tablespoons prepared basil pesto

Instructions:

1.Turn the oven to 200 C. to preheat.

2.Boil vinegar in a saucepan. Lower the heat and simmer until thickened, often whisking, about 15 minutes.

3.In each chicken breast, slice a pocket. Fill an even amount of mozzarella cheese into each pocket and use pepper and salt to season. Wrap 1 ham slice around each chicken breast. In a baking dish, place the wrapped chicken breasts. Around the chicken, put tomatoes and sprinkle olive oil over everything; use pepper and salt to season.

4. Bake for 25 minutes in the preheated oven until the juices run clear and the chicken is no longer pink.

5.Pour a sufficient amount of lightly salted into the saucepan to cover, boil potatoes until soft, about 15 minutes. The strain put back into the pan, and add pesto to coat.

6.On serving dishes, put potatoes, tomatoes, and chicken breasts and drizzle the reduced balsamic vinegar over and enjoy.

Nutrition: Calories 464, Fat 14, Carbs 16, Protein 18, Sodium 620

Pesto Cheesy Chicken Rolls

Prep time: 15 min

Cook time: 50 min

Serve: 2

Ingredients:

- chicken breast

- basil pesto

- cheese

- cooking spray

Instructions:

Set the oven to 175°C to preheat and use cooking spray to coat a baking dish.

Spread onto each flattened chicken breast with 2-3 tbsp. Of pesto sauce, then put over pesto with a slice of cheese. Roll up tightly and use toothpicks to secure, then arrange in a baking dish coated lightly with grease.

In the preheated oven, bake without a cover until juices run clear and chicken is browned beautifully about 45-50 minutes.

Nutrition: Calories 354, Fat 10, Carbs 19, Protein 21, Sodium 389

Chicken Squash Bake

Prep time: 10 min

Cook Time: 30 min

Serve: 2

Ingredients:

- 1 spaghetti squash

- 2 tablespoons olive oil, divided

- 1-1/2 pounds skinless, boneless chicken breast

- salt and ground black pepper to taste

- 1 pinch dried oregano

- 1 pinch garlic powder

- 1 cup pesto

- 1 cup ricotta cheese

- 1 egg yolk

- 1 tablespoon Italian seasoning

- 1 cup marinara sauce

- 1 cup shredded mozzarella cheese

Instructions:

1.Turn the oven to 175°C to preheat.

2.Drizzle over the squash with 1 tablespoon olive oil and put on a cookie sheet with the cut-side turning down.

3.Bake for 20 minutes in the preheated oven until fork-tender. Scrape a fork onto the squash on the inside into spaghetti strands. Evenly spread in a casserole dish.

4.Use garlic powder, oregano, black pepper, and salt to season the chicken breasts.

5.In a big frying pan, heat the leftover 1 tablespoon olive oil over medium heat. Add chicken, cook for 6 minutes each side until turning brown and an instant-read thermometer displays a minimum of 165°F (74°C) when you insert it into the middle.

6.Slice the cooked chicken into half an inch cubes and mix with pesto in a bowl.

7.In a small bowl, mix Italian seasoning, egg yolk, and ricotta cheese.

8.In the casserole dish, top the squash with pesto chicken, ricotta mixture, and 1/2 of the marinara sauce. Make another layer in the same manner. Sprinkle over the top with mozzarella cheese. Put on aluminum foil to cover.

9.Place the preheated oven in the oven and cook for 30 minutes. Until bubbling and the cheese melts. Take away the aluminum foil and broil for 5 minutes until turning golden brown.

Nutrition: Calories 320, Fat 3, Carbs 18, Protein 28, Sodium 520

Pesto Pasta With Chicken

Prep time: 10 min

Cook Time: 30 min

Serve: 2

Ingredients:

- pasta

- olive oil

- garlic

- 2 chicken breasts

- red pepper flakes

- tomatoes

- pesto sauce

Instructions:

1.Boil lightly salted water. Put in pasta and cook till al dente for 8 to 10 minutes; drain.

2.In a big skillet over medium heat, heat oil. Sauté garlic till soft, then mix in chicken. Put red pepper flakes to season. Cook till chicken is golden and cooked through.

3.Put together pesto, sun-dried tomatoes, chicken, and pasta in a big bowl. Coat equally by tossing.

Nutrition: Calories 645, Fat 18, Carbs 32, Protein 36, Sodium 534

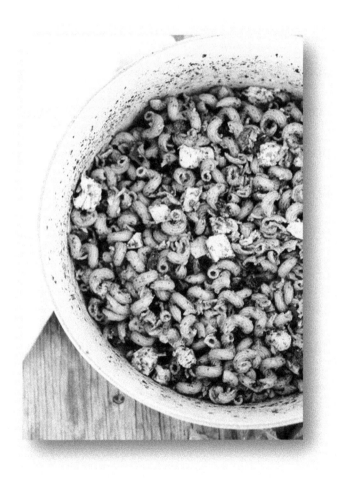

Sheet Pan Chicken With Mozzarella, Pesto, And Broccoli

Prep time: 10 min

Cook Time: 30 min

Serve: 2

Ingredients:

- 2 pounds boneless chicken breasts

- 2 teaspoons garlic salt

- 1 pinch ground black pepper

- 6 tablespoons pesto

- 2 Roma (plum) tomatoes, thinly sliced

- 1 1/2 cups shredded mozzarella cheese

- 1 head broccoli, cut into florets

- 2 tablespoons olive oil

- salt to taste

Instructions:

1.Turn the oven to 425°F to preheat. Lightly coat a big rimmed cookie sheet with oil.

2.On the prepared cookie sheet, put the chicken and sprinkle black pepper and garlic salt over. Spread over the chicken with pesto and put cheese and tomatoes on top.

3.In a bowl, mix oil and broccoli. On the cookie sheet, put broccoli around the chicken. Sprinkle over the top with pepper and salt.

4.Put in the preheated oven and bake for 15-20 minutes until the middle of the chicken is not pink anymore, and the broccoli is soft. An instant-read thermometer should display a minimum of 165°F (74°C) when you insert it into the middle.

Nutrition: Calories 432, Fat 22, Carbs 26, Protein 19, Sodium 455

Chicken Breasts Covered With Parmesan Cheese

Prep time: 5 min

Cook Time: 12 min

Serve: 2

Ingredients:

- ¼ cup panko breadcrumbs

- ¼ cup grated Parmesan cheese

- ¼ tsp. dried basil

- 1 tbsp. olive oil

- 1 tbsp. spicy mustard

- 1 tsp. Worcestershire sauce

- 2 boneless and skinless chicken breasts

Instructions:

1.Put the breadcrumbs, cheese, and basil in a small, shallow bowl. Add and stir the oil until completely mixed. Combine mustard with Worcestershire sauce in a small bowl. Put the mustard mixture on both sides of the breasts.

2. With the crumb mixture, place the chicken in the bowl and press the crumbs on both sides of the breasts to achieve a uniform and firm coating.

3.Put the chicken inside the basket. Cook at a temperature of 185 C. for 21 to 25 minutes, turning halfway through cooking.

Nutrition: Calories 409, Fat 13, Carbs 16, Protein 26, Sodium 534

Chicken in Wheat Cake with Aioli Sauce

Prep time: 10 min

Cook Time: 35 min

Serve: 2

Ingredients:

- 500g breaded chicken

- 4 wheat cakes

- Extra virgin olive oil

- 1 small lettuce

- Grated cheese

- Aioli sauce

Instructions:

1.Put the breaded chicken in the air fryer with a little extra virgin olive oil and fry at 180 degrees for 20 minutes.

2.Take out and reserve.

3.Chop the lettuce, put the wheat cakes on the worktable and distribute the chopped lettuce between them.

4.On the chopped lettuce, spread the pieces of breaded chicken.

5.Cover with grated cheese and add some aioli sauce.

6.Close the wheat cakes and place them on the baking sheet.

7.Take to the oven, 180 degrees, 15 minutes, or until the cheese is melted.

Nutrition: Calories 199, Fat 24, Carbs 21, Protein 18, Sodium 322

Soy Chicken and Sesame, Breaded and Fried

Prep time: 10 min

Cook Time: 25 min

Serve: 2

Ingredients:

- 1 large chicken breast

- Egg

- Breadcrumbs

- Extra virgin olive oil

- Salt

- Ground pepper

- Soy sauce

- Sesame

Instructions:

1.Cut the breast into fillets and put them in a bowl.

2.Season. Add soy sauce and sesame. Flirt well and leave 30 minutes.

3.Beat the eggs and pass all the steaks through the beaten egg and the breadcrumbs.

4.With a silicone brush, permeate the fillets well on both sides.

5.Place on the grill of the air fryer and select 180 degrees, 20 minutes.

6.Make the fillets in batches so that they pile against each other.

Nutrition: Calories 210, Fat 4, Carbs 26, Protein 6, Sodium 534

Chicken with Provencal Herbs and Potatoes

Prep time: 10 min

Cook Time: 55 min

Serve: 2

Ingredients:

- 4 potatoes

- 2 chicken hindquarters

- Provencal herbs

- Salt

- Ground pepper

- Extra virgin olive oil

Instructions:

1.Cut the potatoes into slices after peeling them pepper and put on the grid of the base air fryer.

2.Impregnate the chicken well with oil, salt, and pepper and put some Provencal herbs.

3.Place the chicken on the potatoes.

4.Take the grill to the bucket of the air fryer and put it inside.

5.Select 170 degrees for 40 minutes.

6.Turn the chicken and leave 15 more minutes.

Nutrition: Calories 321, Fat 12, Carbs 21, Protein 21, Sodium 543

Mushroom & Bell Pepper Quiche

Prep Time: 25 minutes

Cook Time: 15 minutes

Serve: 4

Ingredients:

- 6 large eggs
- ½ cup unsweetened almond milk
- Salt and ground black pepper, as required ½ of onion, chopped
- ¼ cup bell pepper, seeded and chopped ¼ cup fresh mushrooms, sliced
- 1 tablespoon fresh chives, minced

Instructions:

1.Preheat your oven to 350 degrees F.

2.Lightly grease a pie dish.

3.In a bowl, add eggs, almond milk, salt, and black pepper and beat until well blended.

4.In a separate bowl, add the onion, bell pepper, and mushrooms and mix.

5.Place the egg mixture into the prepared pie dish evenly and top with vegetable mixture.

6.Sprinkle with chives evenly.

7.Bake for approximately 20-25 minutes.

8.Remove the pie-dish from the oven and set aside for about 5 minutes.

9.Cut into 4 portions and serve immediately.

Nutrition: Calories: 121, Fat: 0g, Carbohydrates: 8g, Fiber: 0.6g, Sugar: 0.1g, Protein: 10g

Green Veggies Quiche

Prep Time: 15 minutes

Cook Time: 20 minutes

Serve: 4

Ingredients:

- 6 eggs
- ½ cup unsweetened almond milk
- Salt and ground pepper, as required 2 cups fresh baby kale, chopped
- ½ cup bell pepper, seeded and chopped 1 scallion, chopped
- ¼ cup fresh parsley, chopped
- 1 tablespoon fresh chives, minced

Instructions:

1. Preheat your oven to 400 degrees F.

2. Lightly grease a pie dish.

3. In a bowl, add eggs, almond milk, salt, and black pepper and beat until well blended. Set aside.

4. In another bowl, add the vegetables and herbs and mix well.

5. In the bottom of the prepared pie dish, place the veggie mixture evenly and top with the egg mixture.

6.Bake for approximately 20 minutes.

7.Remove the pie-dish from the oven and set aside for about 5 minutes before slicing.

8.Cut into desired sized wedges and serve warm.

Nutrition: Calories: 123, Fat: 7.1g, Carbohydrates: 5.9g, Fiber: 1.1g, Sugar: 1.4g, Protein: 9.8g

Zucchini & Carrot Quiche

Prep Time: 10 minutes

Cook Time: 40 minutes

Serve: 3

Ingredients:

- 5 eggs
- Salt and ground black-pepper, as required 1 carrot, peeled and grated 1 small zucchini, shredded

Instructions:

1.Preheat your oven to 350 degrees F.

2.Lightly grease a small baking dish.

3.In a large bowl, add eggs, salt, and black pepper and beat well.

4.Add the carrot and zucchini and stir to combine.

5.Transfer the mixture into the prepared baking-dish evenly.

6.Bake for approximately 40 minutes.

7.Remove the baking-dish from the oven and set aside for about 5 minutes.

8.Cut into equal-sized wedges and serve.

Nutrition: Calories: 119, Fat: 7.4g, Carbohydrates: 3.9g, Fiber: 0.9g, Sugar: 2.2g, Protein: 9.9g

Pineapple Sorbet

Prep Time: 5 min

Cook Time: None

Serve: 4

Ingredients:

- cup mint, fresh

- can pineapple-chunks (1 can = 20oz. in juice, or ½ real pineapple)

Instructions:

1.Wipe the tin or cut the real pineapple and drop it in a freezer bowl (this should freeze for around 2 hours). Keep a few chunks or a loop for garnish.

2.Using a hand blender or food mixer to mix with mint when frozen (keep a few mint leaves aside as well).

3.This seems to work better if you're using fresh pineapple, then we suggest blending first and freezing afterward.

4.When nicely combined, put in bowls and garnish each with the leftover chunks and leaves.

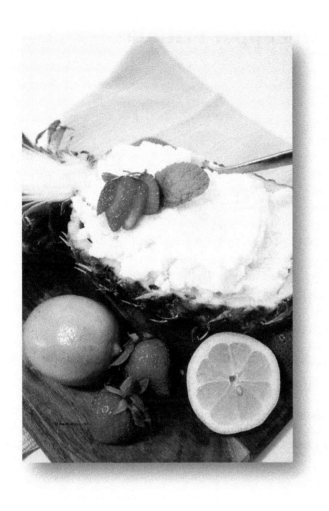

Bell Pepper Frittata

Prep Time: 15 minutes

Cook Time: 10 minutes

Serve: 6

Ingredients:

- 8 eggs
- 1 tablespoon fresh cilantro, chopped
- 1 tablespoon fresh basil, chopped
- ¼ spoon red pepper flakes, crushed Salt, and ground black pepper, as required 2 tablespoons olive oil
- 1 bunch scallions, chopped
- 1 cup bell pepper, seeded and sliced thinly ½ cup goat cheese, crumbled

Instructions:

1.Preheat the broiler of the oven.

2.Arrange a rack in the upper third portion of the oven.

3.In a bowl, add the eggs, fresh herbs, red pepper flakes, salt, and black pepper and beat well.

4.In an ovenproof pan, melt the butter over medium heat and sauté the scallion and bell pepper for about 1 minute.

5.Add the egg mixture over the bell pepper mixture evenly and lift the edges to let the egg mixture flow underneath and cook for about 2-3 minutes.

6.Place the cheese on top in the form of dots.

7.Now, transfer the pan under the broiler and broil for about 2-3 minutes.

8.Removee the pan from the oven and set aside for about 5 minutes before serving.

9.Cut the frittata into desired size slices and serve.

Nutrition: Calories: 167, Fat: 13g, Carbohydrates: 3.3g, Fiber: 0.6g, Sugar: 2.2g, Protein: 9.6g

Zucchini Frittata

Prep Time: 15 minutes

Cook Time: 19 minutes

Serve: 6

Ingredients:

- 2 tablespoons unsweetened almond milk
- 8 eggs
- Salt and ground-black pepper, as required 1 tablespoon olive oil 1 garlic clove, minced
- 2 medium zucchinis, cut into ¼-inch thick round slices ½ cup feta cheese, crumbled

Instructions:

1.Preheat your oven to 350 degrees F.

2.In a bowl, add the almond milk, eggs, salt, and black pepper and beat well. Set aside.

3.In an ovenproof-pan, heat oil over medium heat and sauté the garlic for about 1 minute.

4.Stir in the zucchini and cook for about 5 minutes.

5.Add the egg mixture and stir for about 1 minute.

6.Sprinkle the cheese on top evenly.

7.Immediately transfer the pan into the oven and bake for approximately 10-12 minutes or until eggs become set.

8.Remove the pan from the oveen and set aside to cool for about 3-5 minutes.

9.Cut into desired sized wedges and serve.

Nutrition: Calories: 149, Fat: 11g, Carbohydrates: 3.4g, Fiber: 0.8g, Sugar: 2.1g, Protein: 10g

Chicken & Asparagus Frittata

Prep Time: 15 minutes

Cook Time: 12 minutes

Serve: 4

Ingredients:

- ½ cup cooked chicken, chopped
- ½ cup low-fat Parmesan cheese, grated and divided 6 eggs, beaten lightly
- Salt and ground black-pepper, as required 1/3 cup boiled asparagus, chopped ¼ cup cherry tomatoes, halved

Instructions:

1.Preheat the broiler of the oven.

2.In a bowl, add ¼ cup of the Parmesan cheese, eggs, salt, and black pepper and beat until well blended.

3.In a large oven-proof pan, melt the butter over medium-high heat and cook the chicken and asparagus for about 2-3 minutes.

4.Add the egg mixture and tomatoes and stir to combine.

5.Cook for about 4-5 minutes.

6.Remove from the heeat and sprinkle with the remaining Parmesan cheese.

7.Now, transfer the pan under the broiler and broil for about 3-4 minutes or until slightly puffed.

8.Cut into desired sized wedges and serve immediately.

Nutrition: Calories: 158, Fat: 9.6g, Carbohydrates: 1.6g, Fiber: 0.4g, Sugar: 1g, Protein: 16.2g

Eggs with Spinach

Prep Time: 10 minutes

Cook Time: 22 minutes

Serve: 2

Ingredients:

- 6 cups fresh baby spinach
- 2-3 tablespoons water
- 4 eggs
- Salt and ground black pepper, as required 2-3 tablespoons feta cheese, crumbled

Instructions:

1.Preheat your oven to 400 degrees F.

2.Lightly grease 2 small baking dishes.

3.In a large frying-pan, add spinach and water over medium heat and cook for about 3-4 minutes.

4.Remove the frying pan from heat and drain the excess water completely.

5.Divide the spinach into prepared baking dishes evenly.

6.Carefully crack 2 eggs in each baking dish over spinach.

7.Sprinkle with salt and peppeer and top with feta cheese evenly.

8.Arrange the baking dishes onto a large cookie sheet.

9.Bake for approximately 15-18 minutes.

Nutrition: Calories: 171, Fat: 11.1g, Carbohydrates: 4.3g, Fiber: 2g, Sugar: 1.4g, Protein: 15g

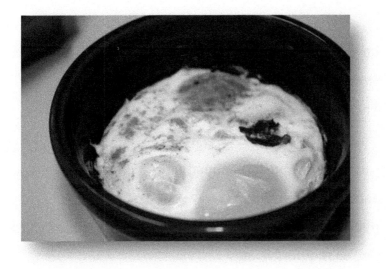

Eggs with Spinach & Tomatoes

Prep Time: 15 minutes

Cook Time: 25 minutes

Serve: 4

Ingredients:

- 2 tablespoons olive oil
- 1 yellow onion, chopped
- 2 garlic cloves, minced
- 1 cup tomatoes, chopped
- ½ pound fresh spinach, chopped
- 1 teaspoon ground cumin
- ¼ spoon red pepper flakes, crushed Salt, and ground black pepper, as required 4 eggs
- 2 tablespoons fresh parsley, chopped

Instructions:

1. In a non-stick pan, heeat the olive oil over medium heat and sauté the onion for about 4-5 minutes.

2. Add the garlic and sauté for approximately 1 minute.

3.Add the tomatoes, spices, salt, and black pepper and cook for about 2-3 minutes, stirring frequently.

4.Add in the spinach and cook for about 4-5 minutes.

5.Carefully crack eggs on top of spinach mixture.

6.With the lid, cover the pan and cook for about 10 minutes.

7.Serve hot with the garnishing of parsley.

Nutrition: Calories: 160, Fat: 11.9g, Carbohydrates: 7.6g, Fiber: 2.6g, Sugar: 3g, Protein: 8.1g

Chicken & Zucchini Muffins

Prep Time: 15 minutes

Cook Time: 15 minutes

Serve: 4

Ingredients:

- 4 eggs
- ¼ cup olive oil
- ¼ cup of water
- 1/3 cup coconut flour
- ½ teaspoon baking powder
- ¼ teaspoon salt
- ¾ cup cooked chicken, shredded
- ¾ cup zucchini, grated
- ½ cup low-fat Parmesan cheese, shredded 1 tablespoon fresh oregano, minced 1 tablespoon fresh thyme, minced
- ¼ cup low-fat cheddar cheese, grated

Instructions:

1.Preheat your oven to 400 degrees F.

2.Lightly greease 8 cups of a muffin tin.

3.In a bowl, add the eggs, oil, and water and beat until well blended.

4.Add the floour, baking powder, and salt, and mix well.

5.Add the remaining ingredients and mix until just blended.

6.Place the muffin mixture into the prepared muffin cup evenly.

7.Bake for approximately 13-15 minutes or until tops become golden brown.

8.Remove muffin tin from oven and place onto a wire rack to cool for about 10 minutes.

9.Invert the muffins onto a platter and serve warm.

Nutrition: Calories: 270, Fat: 20g, Carbohydrates: 3.5g, Fiber: 1.4g, Sugar: 0.9g, Protein: 18g

Turkey & Bell Pepper Muffins

Prep Time: 15 minutes

Cook Time: 20 minutes

Serve: 4

Ingredients:

- 8 eggs
- Salt and ground pepper, as required 2 tablespoons water
- 8 ounces cooked turkey meat, chopped finely
- 1 cup bell pepper, seeded and chopped
- 1 cup onion, finely chopped

Instructions:

1.Preheat your oven to 350 degrees F.

2.Grease 8 cups of a muffin tin.

3.In a bowl, add the eggs, salt, black pepper, and water and beat until well blended.

4.Add the meat, bell pepper, and onion and stir to combine.

5.Place the mixture into the prepared muffin cups evenly.

6.Bake for approximately 17,30-20,30 minutes or until golden brown.

7.Remove the muuffin tin from the oven and place onto a wire rack to cool for about 10 minutes.

8.Carefully invert the muffins onto a platter and serve warm.

Nutrition: Calories: 238, Fat: 11.7g, Carbohydrates: 4.4g, Fiber: 1g, Sugar: 2.5g, Protein: 28.2g

Tofu & Mushroom Muffins

Prep Time: 15 minutes

Cook Time: 30 minutes

Serve: 6

Ingredients:

- 2 teaspoons olive oil, divided
- 1½ cups fresh mushrooms, chopped
- 1 scallion, chopped
- 1 teaspoon garlic, minced
- 1 teaspoon fresh rosemary, minced Freshly ground black pepper, as required
- 1 (12.3-ounce) package lite firm silken tofu, drained ¼ cup unsweetened almond milk
- 2 tablespoons nutritional yeast
- 1 tablespoon arrowroot starch
- ¼ teaspoon ground turmeric

Instructions:

1.Preheat your oven to 375 degrees F.

2.Grease a 12 cups muffin tin.

3.In a non-stick pan, heat 1 spoon of oil over medium heat and sauté scallion and garlic for about 1 minute.

4.Add the mushrooms and sauté for about 5-7 minutes.

5.Stir in the rosemary and black pepper and remove from the heat.

6.Set aside to cool slightly.

7.In a food processor, add the tofu, remaining oil, almond milk, nutritional yeast, arrowroot starch, turmeric, and pulse until smooth.

8.Transfer the tofu mixture into a large bowl.

9.Add the mushroom mixture and gently stir to combine.

10.Move the mixture uniformly into the muffin cups that have been prepared.

11.Bake for 20-22 minutes or until it comes out clean with a toothpick inserted in the center.

12.Remove the mufin tin from the oven and place onto a wire rack to cool for about 10 minutes.

13. Invert the muffins onto the wire rack carefully.

Nutrition: Calories: 70, Fat: 3.6g, Carbohydrates: 4.3g, Fiber: 1.3g, Sugar: 1.1g, Protein: 55.7g

Alkaline Blueberry Spelt Pancakes

Prep Time: 6 minutes

Cook Time: 20 minutes

Serve: 3

Ingredients:

- 2 cups Spelt Flour
- 1 cup Coconut Milk
- 1/2 cup Alkaline Water
- 2 tbsps. Grapeseed Oil
- 1/2 cup Agave
- 1/2 cup Blueberries
- 1/4 tsp. Sea Moss

Instructions:

1. Mix the spelled flour, agave, grapeseed oil, hemp seeds, and sea moss in a bowl.

2. Add in 1 cup of hemp milk and alkaline water to the mixture until you get the consistency mixture you like.

3. Crimp the blueberries into the batter.

4. Heat the skillet to moderate heat, then lightly coat it with the grapeseed oil.

5. Pour the batter into the skillet, then let them cook for approximately 5 minutes on every side.

Nutrition: Calories: 203 kcal Fat: 1.4g Carbs: 41.6g Proteins: 4.8g

Alkaline Blueberry Muffins

Prep Time: 5 Minutes

Cook Time: 20 minutes

Serve: 3

Ingredients:

- 1 cup Coconut Milk
- 3/4 cup Spelt Flour
- 3/4 Teff Flour
- 1/2 cup Blueberries
- 1/3 cup Agave
- 1/4 cup Sea Moss Gel
- 1/2 tsp. Sea Salt
- Grapeseed Oil

Instructions:

1. Adjust the temperature of the oven to 365 degrees.

2. Grease 6 regular-size muffin cups with muffin liners.

3. In a bowl, mix sea salt, sea moss, agave, coconut milk, and flour gel until they are properly blended.

4. You then crimp in blueberries.

5. Coat the muffin pan lightly with the grapeseed oil.

6. Pour in the muffin batter.

7. Bake for at least 30 minutes until it turns golden brown.

Nutrition: Calories: 160 kcal Fat: 5g Carbs: 25g Proteins: 2g

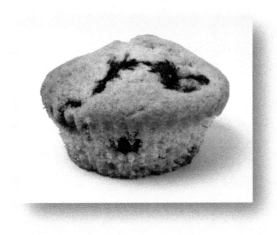

Crunchy Quinoa Meal

Prep Time: 5 minutes

Cook Time: 25 minutes

Serve: 2

Ingredients:

- 3 cups of coconut milk
- 1 cup rinsed quinoa
- 1/8 tsp. ground cinnamon
- 1 cup raspberry
- 1/2 cup chopped coconuts

Instructions:

1. In a saucepan, pour milk and bring to a boil over moderate heat.

2. Add the quinoa to the milk and then bring it to a boil once more.

3. You then let it simmer for at least 15 minutes on medium heat until the milk is reduced.

4. Stir in the cinnamon, then mix properly.

5. Cover it, then cook for 8 minutes until the milk is completely absorbed.

6. Add the raspberry and cook the meal for 30 seconds.

Nutrition: Calories: 271 kcal Fat: 3.7g Carbs: 54g Proteins: 6.5g

25.Coconut Pancakes

Prep Time: 5 minutes

Cook Time: 15 minutes

Serve: 4

Ingredients:

- 1 cup coconut flour
- 2 tbsps. arrowroot powder
- 1 tsp. baking powder
- 1 cup of coconut milk
- 3 tbsps. coconut oil

Instructions:

1. In a medium container, mix in all the dry ingredients.

2. Add the coconut milk and 2 tbsps. Of the coconut oil, then mix properly.

3. Drop a spoon of flour into the skillet and then swirl the pan into a smooth pancake to distribute the batter uniformly.

4. Cook it for like 3 minutes on medium heat until it becomes firm.

5. Turn the pancake to the other side, then cook it for another 2 minutes until it turns golden brown.

6. Cook the remaining pancakes in the same process.

Nutrition: Calories: 377 kcal Fat: 14.9g Carbs: 60.7g Protein: 6.4g

Honey-Lemon Chicken

Prep time: 10 min

Cook Time: 40 min

Serve: 2

Ingredients:

- 2 large chicken thighs

- ½ cup lemon juice

- ¼ cup olive oil

- 1 clove garlic, minced

- 1 teaspoon salt

- ½ teaspoon dried oregano

- 1 Tablespoon honey

- Parsley, chopped, for garnish

Instructions:

1.Preheat broiler (about 450–500°F).

2.Place chicken, skin-side down, in cast iron pan.

3.Broil chicken for 30 minutes, flipping halfway through.

4.While broiling chicken, whisk together lemon juice, olive oil, garlic, salt, and oregano.

5.Brush some of the sauce over the chicken and broil until the chicken (about 3-5 minutes) appears brown and crisp.

6.Transfer skillet to stovetop.

7.Transfer chicken to serving dish, leaving drippings in skillet.

8.Remove any chicken bits from the skillet and drain out any drippings over a couple of tablespoons.

9.Stir in remaining sauce and honey to the skillet.

10.Bring the mixture to a boil and pour over the chicken.

11.Sprinkle with parsley and serve.

Nutrition: Calories 293, Fat 16, Carbs 8, Protein 22, Sodium 432

Greek-Style One Pan Chicken and Rice

Prep time: 5 min

Cook Time: 55 min

Serve: 2

Ingredients:

- 6 chicken thighs

- 2 Tablespoons olive oil, divided

- 1 Tablespoon fresh oregano, chopped

- 1 yellow onion, diced

- 1 cup basmati rice

- 2 cups chicken broth

- ¼ cup of water

- ½ cup cherry tomatoes

- ¼ cup pitted Kalamata olives

- ½–1 lemon, sliced thinly

- Freshly ground black pepper, to taste

- Chopped fresh parsley for garnish

Marinade:

- ¼ cup lemon juice

- Zest of 1 lemon

- 2 Tablespoons fresh oregano, chopped

- 4 cloves garlic, diced

- 1 teaspoon salt

Instructions:

1.Combine marinade ingredients in a shallow container or Ziploc bag.

2.Add the chicken, cover or seal, and let marinate for at least 1 hour to overnight.

3.Preheat oven to 350°F.

4.Heat cast-iron skillet over medium-high heat and swirl in a Tablespoon of oil.

5.Carefully remove the chicken from the marinade (reserving the marinade) and lay skin-side down in the skillet.

6.Cook until the skin is browned (about 3–5 minutes on each side).

7.Transfer chicken to a plate and set aside.

8.Remove any bits of chicken from the skillet and wipe clean with paper towels. (Do this carefully, as the skillet is hot!)

9.Swirl in remaining oil and onion. Cook until onion pieces begin to brown at the edges (about 5 minutes).

10.Stir in the reserved marinade, rice, broth, water, tomatoes, and olives.

11.Bring to a boil.

12.Reduce heat and let simmer briefly (30 seconds).

13.Using a fitted lid or aluminum foil to put chicken on top and cover.

14.Bake for 30 minutes.

15. Remove the lid and put the slices of lemon on top.

16.Bake until chicken is browned and liquid has evaporated (about 10 minutes).

17. Remove from the oven and allow 5-10 minutes to rest.

18.Fluff rice with a fork.

19.Sprinkle with black pepper and chopped parsley, which is freshly ground.

Nutrition: Calories 259, Fat 12, Carbs 10, Protein 18, Sodium 542

Harvest Chicken with Sweet Potatoes, Brussels Sprouts, and Apples

Prep time: 5 min

Cook Time: 35 min

Serve: 2

Ingredients:

- 1 Tablespoon olive oil

- 1 pound boneless, skinless chicken breasts, diced

- 1 teaspoon salt, divided

- ½ teaspoon black pepper

- 4 slices thick-cut bacon, chopped

- 3 cups Brussels sprouts, trimmed and quartered

- 1 medium sweet potato, peeled and diced

- 1 medium onion, chopped

- 2 Granny Smith apples, peeled, cored, and cubed

- 4 cloves garlic, minced

- 2 teaspoons chopped fresh thyme

- 1 teaspoon ground cinnamon

- 1 cup reduced-sodium chicken broth, divided

Instructions:

1.Season chicken with ½ teaspoon salt and pepper.

2.Heat the oil in a cooking pan until it almost starts to sizzle.

3.Add chicken and cook until browned (about 5 minutes).

4.Drain chicken over paper towels and set aside.

5.Reduce heat to medium-low and, using the same skillet, cook bacon until brown and crisp (about 8 minutes).

6.Reserving rendered fat, remove bacon and drain over paper towels.

7.Drain the unnecessary oil / fat from skillet, leaving about 1½ Tablespoons.

8.Add remaining broth and the drained chicken.

9.Let cook through (about 2 minutes).

10.Remove from heat and stir in bacon.

Nutrition: Calories 254, Fat 4, Carbs 26, Protein 6, Sodium 432

Chicken and Vegetable Roast with Dijon Au Jus

Prep time: 35 min

Cook Time: 50 min

Serve: 2

Ingredients:

- 16 fingerling or yellow new potatoes, scrubbed 3 large carrots, cut into 1-inch chunks, divided Salt and pepper, to taste

- 16 Brussels sprouts, halved

- 4 Tablespoons extra-virgin olive oil, divided

- 1 whole 4-pound chicken, cut into 8 serving pieces, backbone reserved 1 cup dry white wine

- 1 whole onion, halved

- 1 stalk celery, roughly chopped

- 3–4 sprigs fresh sage

- 2 bay leaves

- 2 cups low-sodium chicken stock

- 1 medium shallot, sliced thinly

- 2 Tablespoons fresh parsley leaves, minced

- 2 Tablespoons unsalted butter

- 1 Tablespoon Dijon mustard

- Juice of 1 lemon

- 2 teaspoons fish sauce

Instructions:

1.Place potatoes and 2 cups carrot chunks in a saucepan and cover with water. Add about ½ teaspoon of salt and bring to a boil. Let simmer until tender (about 10 minutes). Drain and transfer to a large bowl. Set aside an empty saucepan for later.

2.Add Brussels sprouts to carrots and potatoes. Season with salt and pepper.

3.Add 2 normal spoons olive oil and toss to coat. Set aside.

4.To the saucepan, add the chicken backbone, 1 cup carrots, onion, celery, sage, and bay leaves. Set aside.

5.Preheat oven to 450°F.

6.Clean the parts of chicken with paper towels and season with salt and pepper.

7.Heat 1 spoon oil in a cast-iron skillet over high heat.

8.When oil just begins to smoke, add chicken, skin-side down. Reduce the heat so that the oil does not burn.

9.Cook on the skin-side until golden brown (about 8 minutes), then flip over and brown the other side (about 3 minutes).

10.Transfer chicken to a plate.

11.In the same skillet, pour in white wine. Scrape any brown bits.

12.Carefully transfer white wine from skillet to saucepan with chicken backbone and veggies.

13.Wipe skillet clean.

14.Transfer any juices collected from chicken pieces to a saucepan with backbone and veggies.

15.Pour in chicken stock and bring mixture to a simmer.

16.Reduce heat to the lowest setting, cover, and cook as chicken and other ingredients roast in the oven.

17.Reheat cast iron skillet with remaining oil.

18.When oil just begins to smoke, add potato-carrot-Brussels sprouts mixture and spread evenly.

19.Place chicken pieces, skin-side up, on veggies.

19.Put in the oven e let roast until chicken pieces are done (about 20–45 minutes, with an internal temperature of 150°F for breasts and 165°F for other pieces).

20.Transfer chicken pieces to a serving plate.

21.Add shallot to veggies. Flipping occasionally, roast veggies until browned (about 10 minutes). Remove from the oven.

22.Sprinkle roasted vegetables with parsley and arrange chicken on top.

23.Make the Dijon sauce. Go back to the simmering mixture in the saucepan and drain the broth into a bowl. Whisk in butter, mustard, lemon juice, and fish sauce. Serve the chicken and veggies with the sauce.

Nutrition: Calories 232, Fat 4, Carbs 26, Protein 6, Sodium 645

Cheesesteaks with Chipotle

Prep time: 5 min

Cook Time: 15 min

Serving: 2

Ingredients:

- 1–2 pieces (or to taste) chilies from canned chipotle chilies in adobo sauce, minced 1 Tablespoon adobo sauce

- 2 teaspoons olive oil, divided

- 12 ounces chicken cutlets, sliced thinly

- 1 cup onion, sliced thinly

- 1 cup red bell pepper, pitted and sliced

- 4 cloves garlic, minced

- ¼ teaspoon dried thyme or oregano

- ¼ teaspoon salt

- 1 cup shredded cheddar cheese

- 4 hotdog buns or flour tortillas

- Lime wedges (optional)

Instructions:

1.Heat 1 little spoon oil in a cast-iron skillet over medium-high heat.

2.Sauté chicken until done (about 4–5 minutes). Remove from skillet and set aside.

3.Add remaining oil to the still-hot skillet.

4.Sauté onion, garlic, bell pepper, and thyme/oregano until fragrant and tender (about 4 minutes)

5.Add minced chilies and adobo sauce and let heat through (about 30 seconds).

6.Stir in chicken and season with salt. Cook to heat through (about 1 minute).

7.Remove from heat.

8.Add cheese to the warm mixture and stir to melt.

9.Fill buns or tortillas and serve with lime wedges, if using.

Nutrition: Calories 254, Fat 4, Carbs 26, Protein 6, Sodium 654

Baked Eggs

Prep Time: 10 minutes

Cook Time: 9 minutes

Serve: 6

Ingredients:

- 2 cups fresh spinach, chopped finely
- 12 large eggs
- ½ cup heavy cream
- ¾ cup low-fat Parmesan cheese, shredded Salt and ground black pepper, as required

Instructions:

1.Preheat your oven to 425 degrees F.

2.Grease a 12 cups muffin tin.

3.Divide spinach in each muffin cup.

4.Crack an egg over spinach into each cup and drizzle with heavy cream.

5.Sprinkle with salt and black pepper, followed by Parmesan cheese.

6.Bake for approximately 7-9 minutes or until desired doneness of eggs.

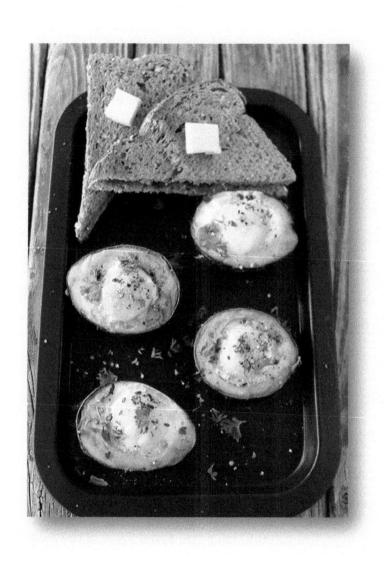

Eggs in Avocado Halves

Prep Time: 10 minutes

Cook Time: 15 minutes

Serve: 2

Ingredients:

- 1 avocado, halved and pitted
- 2 eggs
- Salt and ground black pepper, as required
- ¼ cup cherry tomatoes, halved
- 2 cups fresh baby spinach

Instructions:

1.Preheat your oven to 425 degrees F.

2.Carefully remove about 2 tablespoons of flesh from each avocado half.

3.Place avocado halves into a small baking dish.

4.Carefully crack an egg in each avocado half and sprinkle with salt and black pepper.

5.Bake for about 15 minutes or until the eggs are cooked as desired.

6.Arrange 1 avocado half onto each serving plate and serve alongside the cherry tomatoes and spinach.

Avocado Toast with Eggs

Prep Time: 15 minutes

Cook Time: 4 minutes

Serve: 4

Ingredients:

- 1 large avocado, peeled, pitted, and chopped roughly ¼ teaspoon fresh lemon juice
- Salt and ground pepper, as required 4 whole-wheat bread slices
- 4 boiled eggs, peeled and sliced

Instructions:

1. In a bowl, add the avocado and, with a fork, mash roughly.

2. Add the lemon juice, salt, and black pepper and stir to combine well. Set aside.

3. Heat a nonstick pan on meedium/high heat and toast 1 slice for about 2 minutes per side.

4. Repeat with the remaining slices.

5. Arrange the slices onto serving plates.

6. Spread the avocado mixture over each slice evenly.

7. Top each with egg slices and serve immediately.

Nutrition: Calories: 206, Fat: 13.9g, Carbohydrates: 14g, Fiber: 4.5g, Sugar: 1.4g, Protein: 9.6g

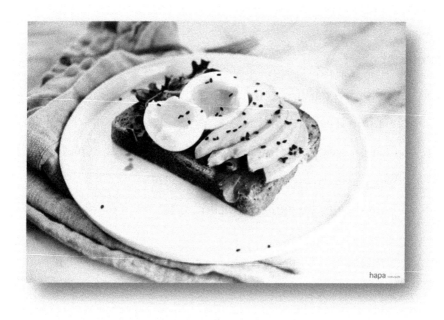

Toast with Egg & Asparagus

Prep Time: 10 minutes

Cook Time: 6 minutes

Serve: 2

Ingredients:

- Olive oil cooking spray
- 10 asparagus spears
- 1 teaspoon olive oil
- 2 large eggs
- 2 large sourdough bread slices, toasted Salt and ground black pepper, as required 1 teaspoon fresh rosemary leaves

Instructions:

1. Heat a griddle pan with cooking spray and heat over high heat.

2. Place the asparagus and cook for about 2-3 minutes per side.

3. Transfer the asparagus onto a plate and drizzle with a little oil.

4. Meanwhile, in a large pan, add the water and a little salt and bring to a boil over high heat.

5. Adjust the heat to low.

6. Carefully crack the eggs in the simmering water and cook for about 3 minutes.

7. With a slotted spoon, transfer the eggs onto a paper towel-lined plate to drain.

8. Divide the bread slices onto serving plates.

9. Top each slice with asparagus spears, followed by 1 egg.

10. Sprinkle with salt and black pepper and serve with the garnishing of rosemary.

Nutrition: Calories: 157, Fat: 7.5g, Carbohydrates: 14g, Fiber: 1.9g, Sugar: 1.9g, Protein: 9.8g

Eggs in Bell Pepper Rings

Prep Time: 10 minutes

Cook Time: 6 minutes

Serve: 2

Ingredients:

- Olive oil cooking spray
- 1 pepper, seeded and cut into 4 (¼-inch) rings
- 4 eggs
- Salt and ground black pepper, as required ¼ teaspoon dried parsley, crushed

Instructions:

1. Heat a nonstick pan with cooking spray and heat over medium heat.

2. Place 4 bell pepper rings in the pan and cook for about 2 minutes.

3. Carefully flip the rings.

4. Crack an egg of each bell pepper ring and sprinkle with salt and black pepper.

5. Cook for about 2-4 minutes or until the desired doneness of eggs.

6. Carefully transfer the bell pepper rings on serving plates and serve with the garnishing of parsley.

Nutrition: Calories: 139, Fat: 8.9g, Carbohydrates: 3.6g, Fiber: 1.1g, Sugar: 2.2g, Protein: 11.7g

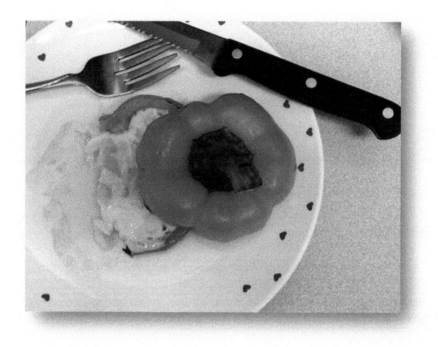

Spinach Waffles

Prep Time: 10 minutes

Cook Time: 20 minutes

Serve: 4

Ingredients:

- 1 large egg, beaten
- 1 cup ricotta cheese, crumbled
- ½ cup part-skim Mozzarella cheese, shredded ¼ cup low-fat Parmesan cheese, grated
- 4 ounces spinach, thawed and squeezed dry
- 1 garlic clove, minced
- Salt and ground black pepper, as required

Instructions:

1. Preheat and then grease the mini waffle iron.

2. Add cheeses, spinach, garlic, salt, and black pepper in a medium mixing bowl and mix until well blended.

3. Place ¼ of the mixture into preheated waffle iron and cook for about 4-5 minutes or until golden brown.

4. Repeat with the remaining mixture.

Nutrition: Calories: 138, Fat: 8.1g, Carbohydrates: 4.8g, Fiber: 0.6g, Sugar: 0.4g, Protein: 11.7g

Kale Scramble

Prep Time: 10 minutes

Cook Time: 6 minutes

Serve: 2

Ingredients:

- 4 eggs
- 1/8 teaspoon ground turmeric
- 1/8 teaspoon red pepper flakes, crushed
- Salt and ground black pepper, as required
- 1 tablespoon water
- 2 teaspoons olive oil
- 1 cup fresh kale, tough ribs removed and chopped

Instructions:

1. In a bowl, add the eggs, turmeric, red pepper flakes, salt, black pepper, and water and beat until foamy.

2. In a pan, heat the oil over meedium heat.

3. Add the egg mixture and stir to combine.

4. Immediately adjust the heat to medium-low and cook for about 1-2 minutes, stirring frequently.

5. Stir the kale in and cook for about 3-4 minutes, stirring frequently.

6.Remove from the heat and serve immediately.

Nutrition: Calories: 183, Fat: 13.4g, Carbohydrates: 4.3g, Fiber: 0.5g, Sugar: 0.7g, Protein: 12.1g

Tomato Scramble

Prep Time: 10 minutes

Cook Time: 5 minutes

Serve: 2

Ingredients:

- 4 eggs
- ¼ spoon red pepper flakes, crushed Salt and ground black pepper, as required ¼ cup fresh basil, chopped ½ cup tomatoes, chopped
- 1 tablespoon olive oil

Instructions:

1.Add the eggs, red pepper flakes, salt, and black pepper in a large bowl and beat well.

2.Add the basil and tomatoes and stir to combine.

3.In a non-stick pan, heat the oil over medium-high heat.

4.Add the egg mixture and cook for about 3-5 minutes, stirring continuously.

Nutrition: Calories: 195, Fat: 15.9g, Carbohydrates: 2.6g, Fiber: 0.7g, Sugar: 1.9g, Protein: 11.6g

Salmon & Arugula Scramble

Prep Time: 10 minutes

Cook Time: 6 minutes

Serve: 4

Ingredients:

- 6 eggs
- 2 tablespoons unsweetened almond milk Salt and ground black pepper, as required 2 tablespoons olive oil
- 4 ounces smoked salmon, cut into bite-sized chunks
- 2 cups fresh arugula, chopped finely
- 4 scallions, chopped finely

Instructions:

1.In a bowl, place the eggs, almond milk, salt, and black pepper and beat well. Set aside.

2.In a non-stick paan, heat the oil over medium heat.

3.Place the egg mixture evenly and cook for about 30 seconds without stirring.

4.Place the salmon, arugula, and scallions on top of the egg mixture evenly.

5.Adjust the heat to low and cok for about 3-5 minutes, stirring continuously.

Nutrition: Calories: 196, Fat: 15g, Carbohydrates: 2g, Fiber: 0.6g, Sugar: 1.1g, Protein: 14g

Apple Omelet

Prep Time: 10 minutes

Cook Time: 9 minutes

Serve: 1

Ingredients:

- 2 teaspoons olive oil, divided
- ½ of large green apple, cored and sliced thinly ¼ teaspoon ground cinnamon 1/8 teaspoon ground nutmeg
- 2 large eggs
- 1/8 teaspoon vanilla extract
- Pinch of salt

Instructions:

1.In a non-stick frying pan, heat 1 spoon of oil over medium-low heat.

2.Add the apple slices and sprinkle with nutmeg and cinnamon.

3.Cook for about 4-5 minutes, turning once halfway through.

4.Meanwhile, in a bowl, add eggs, vanilla extract, and salt and beat until fluffy.

5.Add the reemaining oil to the pan and let it heat completely.

6.Place the egg mixture over apple slices evenly and cook for about 3-4 minutes or until desired doneness.

7.Carefully turn the pan over a serving plate and immediately fold the omelet.

Nutrition: Calories: 258, Fat: 19.5g, Carbohydrates: 9g, Fiber: 1.2g, Sugar: 7g, Protein: 12.8g

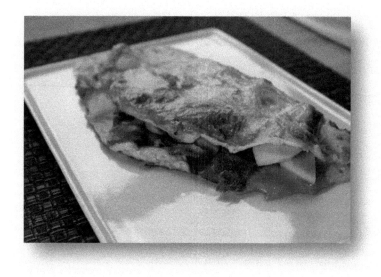

Veggie Omelet

Prep Time: 15 minutes

Cook Time: 15 minutes

Serve: 4

Ingredients:

- 1 teaspoon olive oil
- 2 cups fresh fennel bulb, sliced thinly
- ¼ cup canned artichoke hearts, rinsed, drained, and chopped ¼ cup green olives, pitted and chopped 1 Roma tomato, chopped
- 6 eggs
- Salt and ground black pepper, as required ½ cup goat cheese, crumbled

Instructions:

1.Preheat your oven to 325 degrees F.

2.Heat olive oil in a large ovenprof pan over medium-high heat and sauté the chopped fennel bulb for about 5 minutes.

3.Stir in the artichoke, olives, and tomato and cook for about 3 minutes.

4.Meanwhile, in a bowl, add eggs, salt, and black pepper and beat until well blended.

5.Place the egg mixture over the veggie mixture and stir to combine.

6.Cook for about 2 minutes.

7.Sprinkle with the goat cheese evenly and immediately transfer the pan into the oven.

8.Bake for approximately 5 minutes or until eggs are set completely.

9.Remove the paan from the oven and carefully transfer the omelet onto a cutting board.

10.Cut into desired sized wedges and serve.

Nutrition: Calories: 185, Fat: 12.7g, Carbohydrates: 6.3g, Fiber: 2.3g, Sugar: 1.9g, Protein: 12g

Lightning Source UK Ltd.
Milton Keynes UK
UKHW020651120521
383581UK00005B/54